Prefa[ce]

GW01035564

Get The Airbrush...

As a doctor whose hobby and special interest has ...., ... you will find this booklet helpful. A background knowledge in medical science helped me create these formulas. My clinical knowledge of allergies made me aware of pollutions.

Personally these exercises have amazed me and has helped reduce and almost eliminate the drooping of my eyelids and the down turning at the corners of my month. The exercises for the muscles around the mouth take only two minutes morning and evening. Unlike physical exercises, there is no need to allocate any specific time. You can even carry them out while at work.

Lillysan products on the other hand, gave me that glowing air-brushed look. Best of all, little make up was needed. Remember, that not everybody can afford cosmetic surgery and these exercises can be the alternative. As with all exercises persistence is the key to quicker results. You will be rewarded once you start seeing results.

Remember that women show signs of aging earlier than men. Men don't tend to have that sagging look and their facial lines appear much later. Check out your partners face!
It is now possible to turn back the clock on aging. Nature, pollution, even self inflicted like smoking and changing hormones all take their toll on your face. Follow these simple instructions in the booklet and take control of your face and the aging process. It is simple and priceless.

Lillysan cosmetic Ingredients are well known anti-aging products found in most anti-aging creams, but with the right concentration, results are visible within weeks of use. Don't let this chance pass you by, exercise your face and use these amazing products.

Take control of your face.

Dr. S. L. Gravenir

Section 1

General Notes on the Skin

ANATOMY OF SKIN

The Skin has three main layers. The **hypodermis** is the lower layer of skin. This is composed of muscle and fatty tissue and differs from person to person, more thicker in women, hence the rounded female face.

Severe dieting has a negative effect on the hypodermis, thereby losing the fatty tissue and appearing gaunt. Likewise, an overweight person appears more youthful.

The **dermis** is the layer above the hypodermis and is made up of connective tissue, mainly collagen and elastin. The outer skin layer is the **epidermis**. It is made of two layers, the **living basal layer** which is next to the hypodermis and **stratum corneum** which is composed of dead keratin – filled cells. Melanocyes, responsible for skin colour are found in the basal cells . Basal cells are constantly being renewed becoming flatter, losing their moisture and are shed as dead skin cells. The dead skin should be removed regularly as these give the skin a dull appearance.

This forms the basis of routine exfoliation of skin. The least expensive method of exfoliation is by using a muslin cloth to dry rub the face once a week.

As we age the skin loses its elasticity because production of collagen diminishes. However, the skin is very permeable to topical creams and serums. For the skin to start renewing the production of collagen, the creams and serums have to contain the proper ingredients in high content or percentages for good results.

What is Collagen?

Collagen is a protein found in animal connective tissue. It is one of the building blocks and is made of different amino acids. Collagen gives the skin elasticity and strength. Loss of collagen as you age contributes to the visible signs of aging. There are twenty nine types of collagen. Collagen C and Hyaluronic Acid are two of the most important in the aging process. As production of collagen decreases, so does the appearance of fine lines and wrinkles which become more visible. Collagen cannot be applied topically on skin because the molecules are large and will not penetrate the skin. Therefore it is important to eat food rich in Collagen to replenish the depleted supplies.

Collagen Rich Foods

The following are examples of Collagen rich foodstuffs:

Soy Products:
Soya Milk, Soya cheese, both contain a natural plant hormone which increases the production of Collagen.

Red Fruits and Vegetables:
All coloured foods have anti-oxidant properties. Red apples, red berries, strawberries, beetroot and red peppers and red potatoes. Try and include any of these in your daily diet.

Beans, Sprouts and Cabbage:
Carrots – A very good source of Vitamin A which is known to slow down the breakdown of Collagen and Elastin. Vitamin A thickens and stimulates the dermis.

Nuts:
Walnuts and flaxseeds all contain Omega 3 fatty acids. These are so called essential oils which the body cannot produce.

Olives:
Both black and green olives are rich in Sulphur which is known to promote Collagen production.

Lemons and Oranges:
Both contain Vitamin C, a well known anti-oxidant which help Collagen production. The body cannot produce or store Vitamin C, so it is important to eat these fruits every

day. Vitamin C has many other properties.

Avocados:
Avocados contain plant steroids which can reduce age spots. They also contain Vitamin E (another anti-oxidant) and Omega 3 fatty acids.

Turkey:
"Not only for Christmas" Turkey meat and skin have a particular amino acid, carnosine which reduces skin aging. Turkey meat also contains Zinc. Zinc promotes Collagen and skin cell growth. Zinc also reduces skin inflammation and boosts the immune system.

Facial Treatments For Problem Skin - Facts

Dull Skin
Glowing skin is a sign of youth. Babies, children and young people have it. However, as we age the skin begins to appear dull. This is a result of reduced new cell turn over. Once you reach a certain age, you need to start looking after your face. There is regular **exfoliating, chemical peels** and **spa or expert peels.**
At home peels are those bought in your local pharmacy. These are very mild and the result at most is minimal. Spa peels have higher levels of the acid (glycolic, salicylic lactic and trichloroacetic acids) than you're at home peels. It is best to use these not more than twice a month.

Expert peels carried out by your dermatologist have different strengths or percentage of the acids. 20% of the acids would be a mild peel and 99% of the acids would be deep peel. Mild peels can be applied once a week, while medium and deep peels can cause some skin irritation. Your dermatologist should be able to advice. Remember to wear a good sunscreen after the peels.

Loss of Elasticity
As we age, your skin loses its elasticity most noticeable on your face. It gets worse after

menopause. Smoking, sun exposure stress and poor diet can all decrease skin elasticity.

Laser skin rejuvenation is the latest in skin elasticity. However, it can be expensive. High intensity of light pulses is applied to the skin surface. The skin later heals itself by producing more elastic new collagen. It takes up to five treatments with three to four weeks intervals. The skin will appear more toned and the complexion will be more even.

Brown Spots, Age Spots and Sun Spots

These spots become more permanent as we age. There are results of many factors, genetics, and exposure to sunlight without protection, hormonal changes in pregnancy and at menopause. There are creams available to reduce the amount of *melanin* that is produced. The creams contain a skin bleaching chemical containing *hydroquinone*. Over the counter creams contain only 2% of Hydroquinone, 4% Hydroquinone is by prescription only.

The best way to remove these spots is by *laser skin resurfacing*. Stubborn spots may just fade. Remember that your body continues to produce melanin. So it is better to keep away from the sun or wear sun protection. All these procedures are expensive.

Skin Toning by Non Surgical Face Lift

Acupuncture Facial

Tiny needles are inserted into specific spots on the face and scalp. The needles cause the facial muscles to contract and relax. A course of up to 12 weekly sessions is required before any change can be noticed.

Thermage

Radio frequency is required to tighten and tone the skin. Heat created by the radio frequency causes the collagen to tighten. Thermage is best for those with slight losses of elasticity and minimal sagging. You will need monthly treatments for six months. Treatments maybe expensive.

Titan

This is another laser light therapy using infra red light which heats the dermis. The collagen then contracts and tightens. It also encourages growth of new, more elastic collagen. You will need up to six of monthly treatments.

PS: These are very expensive procedures, which not everybody can afford.

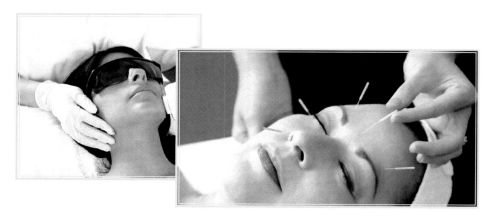

Section 2

Notes on Facial Muscles and Facial Anatomy

The muscles of the face are attached directly to the skin that covers them. So when the facial muscles sag the skin attached to them also sag. The sagging of the muscles and skin leads to the well known drooping of the upper eyelids, bags under the eyes and turkey necks.

The muscles on your face as illustrated can be exercised with amazing results. With regular exercise cheeks will become plumper, lines on your upper lip will decrease, the corners of your mouth will become firmer and lines above your upper lip will decrease; neck and jaw line will become firmer. The results are evident within three months.

The circular muscles around the eyes called Orbicularis Oculi tend to sag as we age. Thereby causing drooping of the eyelids. Likewise, there are circular muscles around the mouth aptly called Orbicularis Oris which also tend to sag as we age. This causes drooping of the lower lip and combined with weakened Depresser anguli oris results in the classical down turning at the corners of the mouth.

At a glance of the facial muscles, you can see which muscles needs toning by these regular exercises.

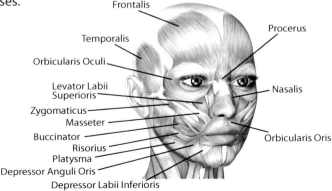

Section 3

Facial Exercises

We all know about triceps, biceps, pectoralis and rectus abdominis. These are all muscles routinely exercised by everyone who want to achieve that body. We tend to forget about our facial muscles.

These muscles have to be exercised as well to stop the natural process of aging resulting in sagging of the face. The sagging is worse for women than men, most probably due to hormonal changes.

The exercises are usually very easy to carry out. Each person can decide on which muscles to concentrate on. Target the muscles which you feel need more toning and exercise them. Know your problem facial muscles.

If you have the usual down turning of the lower lips, then exercise the muscle orbiculari Oris. Likewise, if you're upper lids are drooping target the orbicularis oculi. Check the photographs and concentrate on the exercises which suit you. Three minutes twice a day is all you need and the results can be seen within a month or two.

You do not need to allocate any special time for these exercises; they can be carried out while sitting at your desk or just before falling asleep at night. I carry out mine just before getting out of bed in the morning and last thing before falling asleep.

Remember that you are judged by your looks as the looks form the very first impression of who you are. So look after your face. You appear and feel as young as you look.

In the next few pages, I will demonstrate the actual exercises you can do. The best ones which are starred give the best results.

To Improve Sagging of the Corners of the Mouth

- Place your lower lip over the upper lip, tensing the corners of your mouth and tilting your head back.

- You are doing well when you feel the tension around your cheeks.

- You should feel your neck stretching and tension around your mouth.

- Hold this to a count of ten.

- Relax.

- Repeat up to six times.

- Do this twice a day. Best time is before getting up in the morning and last thing at night before bed. It Is all about toning and since facial muscles are thinner, less time is needed for exercising.

- Make these exercises a daily routine. Missing a day is ok.

- It is all about toning and since facial muscles are thinner less time is needed for exercising.

To Improve Drooping of the Upper Eyelids

- Curve your 5th finger under your eyebrows.

- Hold each side of your head with your thumbs.

- Push up your eyebrows firmly and close your eyes slowly, you will feel a good downwards pull.

- Now squeeze your eyelids really tightly and hold for a count of ten.

- Open your eyes relax and breathe.

- Repeat six times.

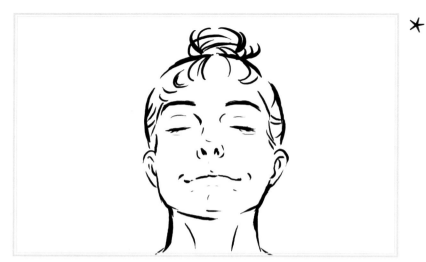

To Improve Sagging of the Corners of the Mouth

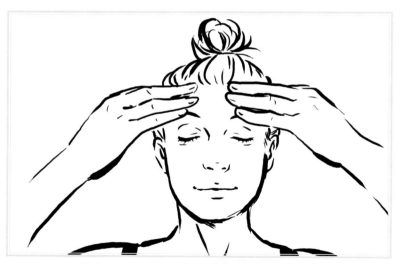

To Improve Drooping of the Upper Eyelids

To Erase Lines on the Upper Lips

I find this exercise best done in the shower; which makes the movements easier.

• Place your thumbs under your upper lip in the midline position.

• Make sure your upper lip grasp your thumbs firmly.

• Move your thumbs sideways towards the corners of your mouth. Feel the pull.

• Repeat ten times.

To Strengthen the Lips and the Surrounding Muscles

• Open your mouth as if yawning.

• Lower your lower jaw in slow movements, moving the corners of your mouth slowly inwards.

• Your mouth should form an oval shape.

• The muscles around your mouth should feel taut; remember to draw your jaw as low as possible.

• Hold and count up to 10. Relax. *(Repeat x6 times)*.

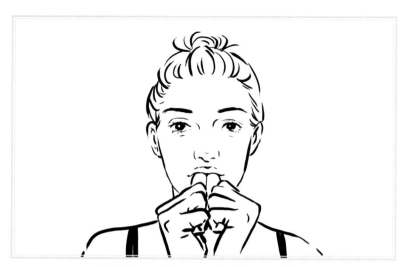

To Erase Lines on the Upper Lips

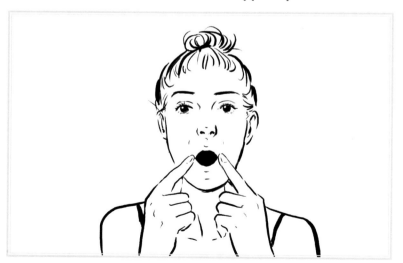

To Strengthen the Lips and the Surrounding Muscles

To Exercise the Muscles of the Neck and Jaw Line

- Sit comfortably.

- Tilt your head up and back slightly, the sniffing position, and lift out your chin.

- Keep your head still; open your mouth wide by lowering your jaw.

- Bring your back teeth gently together. Still grinning, lower and raise your jaw ten times.

- Notes: Keep the grin throughout. Relax your forehead and you should feel no tension in your eye area.

To Firm the Muscles under the Chin and Help Eliminate a Double Chin

- Hold your chin in a sniffing position.

- Place your elbows on a firm surface and place your clenched fist under your chin.

- Place your bottom lip over your upper lip.

- Press the tip of your tongue against the roof of your mouth.

- Hold this position for five seconds.

- Slowly release the pressure, slowly counting to five.

- Relax. *(Repeat x6 times)*.

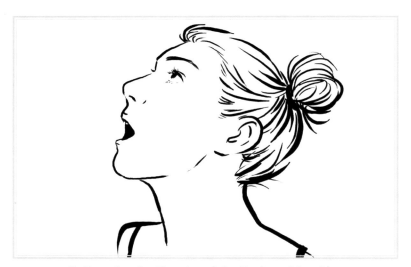

To Exercise the Muscles of the Neck and Jaw Line

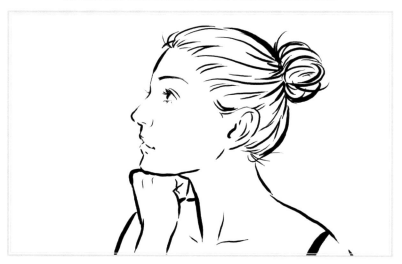

To Firm the Muscles under the Chin and Help Eliminate a Double Chin

To Prevent and Help Eliminate Scowl Lines

• Stand in front of a mirror as before.

• (Place the palm of your hand over the eyebrows to hold them still).

• Close your eyes and look down.

• Count up to ten. Then release in slowly.

• Relax.

• Repeat x 6. Repeat this several times a day.

To Eliminate Lines on the Bridge of the Nose

• Place your thumbs on each side of your face.

• Place your third fingers on the top of the bridge of your nose.

• Now move your fingers over the muscles in an up and down fashion in five tiny slow movements.

• Hold for five seconds.

• Slowly relax. Repeat x 3.

• PS. DO NOT SCOWL.

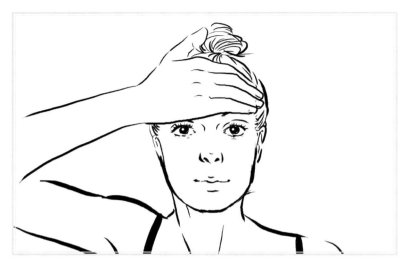

To Prevent and Help Eliminate Scowl Lines

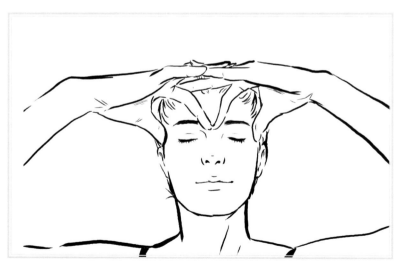

To Eliminate Lines on the Bridge of the Nose

Section 4

Lillysan Products ~ Lillysan Serum

Lillysan Serum contains mainly Glycoaminoglycan which has amazing moisturizing effect on skin and is also known as Natural Moisturizing factor. Glycoaminoglycan can absorb up to 1000 x its weight in water. A super moisturiser, in simple language. Glycoaminoglycan is mostly found in collagen.

Gycosaminoglycan forms a gel that cushions jowls and nerves, fills eyes and plumps skin. It has a well known plumping effect. However as we age, the production of Glycoaminoglycan slows which results in more pronounced wrinkles.

When applied to skin, the Glycoaminoglycan forms a thin layer keeping the skin smooth and moist; and penetrates into deep layers to eliminate wrinkles and increasing elasticity.

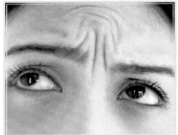

GAG is the most powerful hydrator currently available on the market. It is important to use a good sun cream after the Glycoaminoglycan. The effects are visible within two weeks of use. Apply serum to cleansed damp skin to lock in the moisture twice a day. Remember to apply over the neck region. All other creams have to be applied after, an interval of ten minutes so as to avoid dilution of the Glycoaminoglycan.

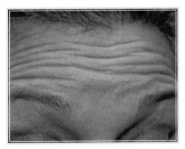

You can use Lillysan cream after fifteen minutes to lock in the serum. It is important to use SPF 50 everyday even on overcast rainy days, as Glycoaminoglycan can increase skins sensitivity to sunlight. The serum is best for crow's feet (laughter lines) and wrinkles around the mouth caused by smoking and age.

The overall result is that of a plumping effect.

Lillysan Cream

Creme De La Creme

One of the two main ingredients of this cream is from a marine extract. It has an anti-inflammatory and anti- itch activities. It is used as a base in the cream for its moisturizing pr operties.

The cream also contains other ingredients which improve the firmness of the skin and helps to reduce the visible appearance of sagging skin when used twice a day, results are evident from two weeks of use. This cream would suit those with sagging skin especially around the mouth.

People suffering from Rosacea and broken facial veins will also benefit from the cream. The cream also forms the base for aftershave cream.

Lillysan Cream complements the Lillysan Serum.
When using both, apply the serum first, then the cream about fifteen minutes later. Pat the serum and cream onto your face, do not rub them in. A very small amount is needed. Remember less is more.

Those ordering Lillysan cream for Rosacea, broken facial veins and aftershave skin reactions should specifically ask for Lillysan Cream S.

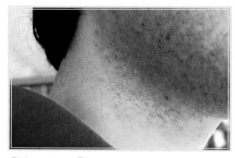

Aftershave Reactions

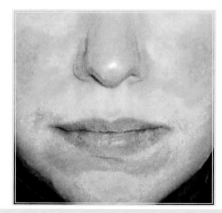

Lillysan Vitamin C Serum

Vitamin C is anti-aging and reverses sun damage. It's a powerful anti oxidant and it protects against environmental damage and rejuvenates collagen fibres. It also provides sun protection, lightens skin pigmentation, therefore important with people with different skin tones.

It takes about four weeks of continued use to start seeing benefits, your skin will appear more youthful and your friends will start noticing the difference. It is important to stress that Vitamin C may make you be more sensitive to sunlight, therefore it is important to wear a good sun cream of up to 50 SPF sun cream.

Vitamin C is one of the best ingredients for the production of collagen when applied topically. It is Important to note that Vit C is unstable when exposed to air and light. Therefore it should be stored in the fridge away from direct light. Vitamin C is a powerful anti-oxidant and production of collagen starts within six weeks of use. Vitamin C serum can be used by all age groups.

The body cannot store Vitamin C which is found in most fruits, so in order to get enough Vitamin C you will need to consume large quantity of fruits every day, but this is not practical.

Vitamin C Serum also targets brown age spots and uneven skin tones. Results are visible (if applied twice daily) within six weeks. Vitamin C Serum brightens the skin giving it a healthy glow. For best and quick results, apply twice a day.
Vitamin C promotes the absorption of Glycoaminoglycan in Lillysan Serum.
Vitamin C serum can be used by people of Asian and African origins who tend to have uneven skin tones, especially around the eyes.

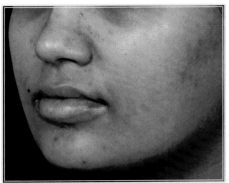

Lillysan Eye Cream

The eye cream was especially formulated to target deep crow's feet around the eyes, the area around the eyes is very delicate. The subcutaneous tissue in this region is very thin and shows signs of aging earlier. Apply a thin layer of cream on affected areas; literally pat a tiny amount of cream preferably before going to bed. Results can be seen the next day.

The eye cream is best for stubborn wrinkles around the eyes. Avoid application over upper and lower eyelids.

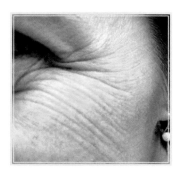 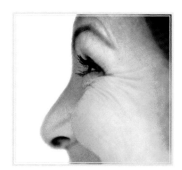

Lillysan Neck Cream

The area around the neck and the décolletage region have thin subcutaneous tissue. So if you are of normal or average weight, these areas show earlier signs of aging. These areas are exposed to the adverse effects of the sun and of alcohol from perfumes which are normally sprayed over these regions. Lillysan neck cream targets the décolletage and neck regions.

Tip: Do not spray your favourite perfume over these regions.

PS: Lillysan Eye Cream and Lillysan Neck Cream are rescue remedies for those with visible wrinkles and those who want a quick fix. If you use both Lillysan Serum and Cream regularly, you may not need the Eye and Neck Creams, depending on your age.

Section 5

A-Z in Skin Care

- *Alpha Hydroxy acids (AHAS)*, there are naturally occurring acids which clear surface dead skin cells and which speed up the natural exfoliation process. AHAS are available naturally in dairy products (lactic acid) sugar (glycolic acid) and citric fruits (citric acid). AHAS reduces fine lines and help in cleaning pores. They are normally used in peels. Careful if you have sensitive skin.

- *Antioxidants*, they protect the skin from damaging free radicals (oxidants). The so called free radicals are unstable molecules as a result of pollution, smoke, UV light and other pollutions. Free radicals can attack the skin and cause visible signs of aging. Examples of antioxidants are Vitamin C, Vitamin E and green tea.

- *Ceramides* help prevent water loss. They encourage skin cell renewal. These are ingredients in moisturisers which are first line defence in dry cracked and chapped skin.

- *Collagen*, A well known protein found naturally in young skin. There is controversy whether creams with collagen actually boost the skins ability to produce collagen. Vitamin C has been known to promote the production of collagen. You will need to consume vast quantity of vitamin C as the body cannot store any excess.

- *Glycolics* , Are part of alpha hydroxy acids which speed up the shedding of dead cells.

- *Growth Factors*, These are used in anti aging cream to help build collagen and soften wrinkles. TNS recovering complex is an example of a growth factor.

- *Hyaluronic Acid*, A sugar molecule used in many moisturisers because it has the ability to attract water, thereby reducing fine lines and wrinkles.

- *Hydroquinone*, it's an oxidant which also suppresses the enzymes in the skin that are responsible for melanin production. They lighten age spots and dark spots.

- *Retinoids* are Vitamin A derivatives that help collagen production. They have been used in the treatment of acne. **Topical Retin A** and **Renova creams** are examples. They are available on prescriptions only. Not suitable for sensitive skin. **Soy Isoflavones** are so called plant oestrogens can block melanin production and thereby reduce the appearance of dark spots. They may also prevent collagen loss in post menopausal women due to their oestrogen properties.

Other Tips

- Use non alcoholic wipes.

- Do not spray perfume over the décolletage region, the alcohol in the perfume dries the skin and causes wrinkles.

- Hydrate your skin by drinking enough water.

- Exfoliate your face up to three times a week using a mild soft scrub.

Notes

Notes